The Ultimate Sous Vide Cookbook

60 Most wanted Recipes with detailed Techniques and Instruction for Busy People. Lose Weight Fast and start cook like a pro in a few steps

Frank Kimmons

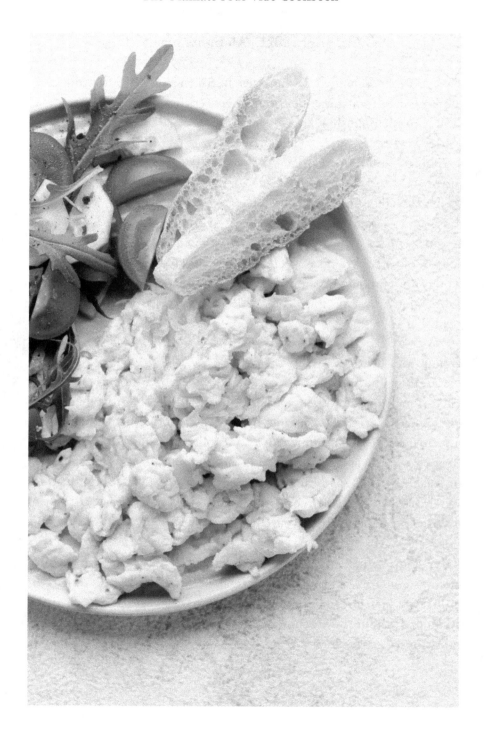

Table of Contents

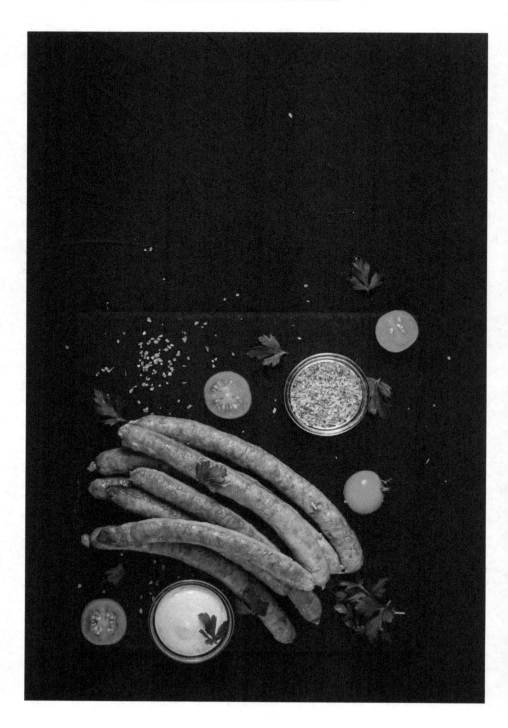

CHAPTER 1.   Red Meats

1. Tamari Steak with Scramble Eggs

Prep + Cook Time: 1 hour 55 minutes | Servings: 4

Ingredients

- ¼ cup milk
- 1 cup Tamari sauce
- ½ cup brown sugar
- ⅓ cup olive oil
- 4 garlic cloves, chopped
- 1 tsp onion powder
- Salt and black pepper to taste
- 2 ½ pounds skirt steak
- 4 eggs

Directions

Prepare a water bath and place the Sous Vide in it. Set to 130 F. Combine the Tamari sauce, brown sugar, oil, onion powder, garlic, sea salt and pepper. Place the steak in a vacuum-sealable bag with the mixture. Release air by the water displacement method, seal, and submerge the bag in the water bath. Cook for 1 hour and 30 minutes.

In a bowl, combine eggs, milk, and salt. Stir well. Scramble the eggs in a skillet over medium heat . Set aside. Once the timer has stopped, remove the steak and pat it dry. Heat a skillet over high heat and sear the steak for 30 seconds per side. Cut into tiny strips. Serve with the scrambled eggs.

2. Tasty Short Ribs with BBQ Sauce

Prep + Cook Time: 12 hours 15 minutes | Servings: 4

Ingredients

- 2 tbsp butter
- 1 ½ pounds beef short ribs
- Salt and black pepper to taste
- 3 tbsp toasted sesame oil
- 1 ½ cups barbecue sauce
- 10 garlic cloves, smashed
- 3 tbsp champagne vinegar 2 tbsp minced fresh ginger
- ⅛ cup chopped scallions
- ⅛ cup sesame seeds

Directions

Prepare a water bath and place the Sous Vide in it. Set to 186 F. Season the ribs with salt and pepper. Heat sesame oil in a skillet over high heat and sear each rib for 1 minute per side. Combine the BBQ sauce, garlic, vinegar, and ginger. Place three ribs in each vacuumsealable bag with the BBQ sauce. Release air by the water displacement method, seal, and submerge the bag in the water bath. Cook for 12 hours.

Once the timer has stopped, remove the ribs and pat dry with kitchen towel. Heat a saucepan over medium heat and pour the cooking juices. Cook for 4-5 minutes until sticky. Heat the butter in a skillet over high heat and sear the ribs for 1 minute per side. Top with the BBQ sauce. Garnish with scallions and sesame seeds.

3. Caribbean Chili Steak Tacos

Ready in about 2 hours 10 minutes | Servings: 4

Ingredients

- 1 tbsp canola oil
- 2 pounds flank steak
- Salt and black pepper to taste
- 1 tsp garlic powder
- 2 tsp lime juice
- Zest of 1 lime
- Zest and juice of 1 orange
- 1 tsp red pepper flakes
- 1 garlic clove, minced
- 1 tbsp butter
- 12 corn tortillas
- 1 head red cabbage, sliced
- Pico de gallo, for serving
- Sour cream, for serving
- 4 serrano peppers, sliced

Directions

Prepare a water bath and place the Sous Vide in it. Set to 130 F. Season the steak with salt, pepper and garlic powder. Combine the lime juice and zest, orange juice and zest, red pepper flakes, and garlic. Place the steak and the sauce in a vacuum-sealable bag. Release air by the water displacement method. Refrigerate for 30 minutes. Seal and submerge into the water bath. Cook for 90 minutes. Once the timer has stopped, remove the steak and pat dry with kitchen towels. Heat the oil and the butter in a skillet over high heat and sear the steak for 1 minute.Cut the steak into slices. Fill the tortilla with the steak. Garnish with cabbage, pico de gallo, sour cream and serrano.

Serve and enjoy!

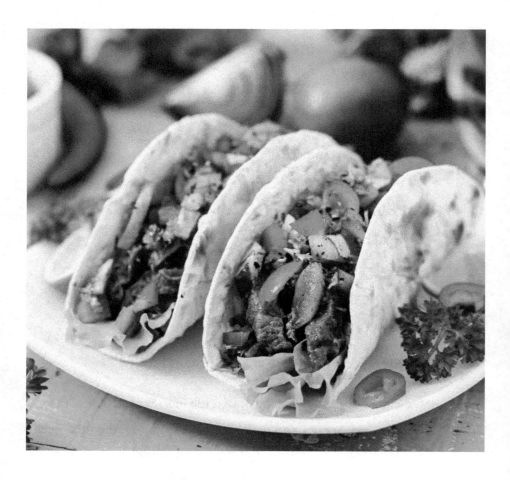

4. Chili Beef Tenderloin

Prep + Cook Time: 3 hours 20 minutes | Servings: 4

Ingredients

- 2 tbsp ghee
- 2 ¼ pounds beef tenderloin
- Salt and black pepper to taste
- 1 tbsp chili oil
- 2 tsp dried thyme
- 1 tsp garlic powder
- ½ tsp onion powder
- ½ tsp cayenne pepper

Directions

Prepare a water bath and place the Sous Vide in it. Set to 134 F. Season the tenderloin with salt and pepper. Combine the chili oil, thyme, garlic powder, onion powder, and cayenne pepper. Brush the mixture over the tenderloin. Place the tenderloin in a vacuum-sealable bag. Release air by the water displacement method, seal, and submerge the bag in the water bath. Cook for 3 hours.

Once the timer has stopped, remove the tenderloin and pat dry with a kitchen towel. Heat the ghee in a skillet over high heat and sear the tenderloin for 45 seconds per side. Allow to rest for 5 minutes. Cut it and serve.

5. Saucy Beef Sirloin

Prep + Cook Time: 1 hour 50 minutes | Servings: 6

Ingredients

- 2 tbsp olive oil
- 3 pounds beef sirloin, cut into strips
- Salt and black pepper to taste
- 2 tbsp white wine vinegar
- ½ tbsp freshly squeezed lemon juice
- 1 tsp allspice
- ½ tbsp garlic powder
- onion, chopped
- 1 tomato, chopped
- 2 garlic cloves, minced
- tbsp soy sauce
- cups cooked quinoa

Directions

Prepare a water bath and place the Sous Vide in it. Set to 134 F. Season sirloin with salt and pepper. Combine well 1 tbsp of olive oil, white wine vinegar, lemon juice, allspice, and garlic powder. Mix together the sirloin with the marinade and place it in a vacuumsealable bag. Release air by the water displacement method, seal, and submerge the bag in the water bath. Cook for 1 hour and 30 minutes.

Meanwhile, heat the olive oil in a saucepan over medium heat and stir in onion, tomato, garlic, and soy sauce. Cook for 5 minutes until the tomato begins to soften. Set aside. Once the timer has stopped, remove the sirloin and pat dry with kitchen towel. Reserve the cooking juices. Heat a skillet over high heat and sear for 1-2 minutes.

Combine the cooking juices with the tomato mix. Cook for 4-5 minutes until simmer. Add in sirloin and stir for 2 minutes more. Serve with quinoa.

6. Fire-Roasted Tomato Tenderloin

Prep + Cook Time: 2 hours 8 minutes | Servings: 4

Ingredients

- 2 pounds center-cut beef tenderloin, 1-inch thick
- 1 cup fire-roasted tomatoes, chopped
- Salt and black pepper to taste
- 3 tbsp of extra virgin olive oil
- 2 bay leaves, whole
- 3 tbsp of butter, unsalted

Directions

Prepare a water bath, place Sous Vide in it, and set to 136 F. Thoroughly rinse the meat under the running water and pat dry with paper towels. Rub well with the olive oil and generously season with salt and pepper. Place in a large vacuum-sealable bag along with fireroasted tomatoes and two bay leaves.

Seal the bag, submerge in the water bath and cook for 2 hours. Once done, remove the bags, place the meat on a baking sheet. Discard the cooking liquid. In a large skillet, melt the butter over medium heat. Add the tenderloin and sear for 2 minutes on each side. Serve with your favorite sauce and vegetables.

7. Soy Garlic Tri-Tip Steak

Prep + Cook Time: 2 hours 5 minutes | Servings: 2

Ingredients

- 1 ½ lb tri-ip steak
- Salt and black pepper to taste
- 2 tbsp soy sauce
- 6 cloves garlic, roasted and crushed

Directions

Make a water bath, place Sous Vide in it, and set to130 F. Season the steak with pepper and salt and place it in a vacuum-sealable bag. Add in the soy sauce. Release air by the water displacement method and seal the bag. Submerge in the water bath and set the timer for 2 hours. Once the timer has stopped, remove and unseal the bag. Heat a pan over high heat, place the steak in and sear on both sides for 2 minutes each. Slice and serve in a salad.

8. Greek Meatballs with Yogurt Sauce

Prep + Cook Time: 1 hour 10 minutes | Servings: 4

Ingredients

- 1 pound lean ground beef
- ¼ cup bread crumbs
- 1 large egg, beaten
- 2 tsp fresh parsley
- Sea salt and black pepper to taste 3 tbsp extra-virgin olive oil
- Yogurt Sauce:
- 6 ounces Greek yogurt
- 1 tbsp extra-virgin olive oil
- Fresh dill
- Lemon juice from 1 lemon
- 1 garlic clove, minced
- Salt to taste

Directions

Start with the preparation of yogurt sauce. Whisk together all sauce ingredients in a medium bowl, cover and refrigerate for 1 hour. Prepare a water bath, place Sous Vide in it, and set to 141 F. Place the meat in a large bowl. Add the beaten egg, bread crumbs, fresh parsley, salt, and pepper. Thoroughly combine the ingredients together. Shape bite-sized balls and place in a large vacuum-sealable bag in a single layer.

Seal the bag and cook in a water bath for 1 hour. With a slotted spoon, carefully remove from the bag and discard the cooking liquid. Sear the meatballs in a medium-hot skillet with olive oil until they are browned, 2-3 minutes per side. Top with yogurt sauce and serve.

9. Dijon & Curry Ketchup Beef Sausages

Prep + Cook Time: 1 hour 45 minutes | Servings: 4

Ingredients

- ½ cup Dijon mustard
- 4 beef sausages
- ½ cup curry ketchup

Directions

Prepare a water bath and place the Sous Vide in it. Set to 134 F.

Place the sausages in a vacuum-sealable bag. Release air by the water displacement method, seal, and submerge the bag in the water bath. Cook for 90 minutes. Once the timer has stopped, remove the sausages and transfer to a high heat grill. Cook for 1-3 minutes until the grill marks appear. Serve with mustard and curry ketchup.

10.Lamb Chops with Basil Chimichurri

Prep + Cook Time: 3 hours 40 minutes | Servings: 4

Ingredients

- <u>Lamb Chops:</u>
- 3 lamb racks, frenched
- 3 cloves garlic, crushed Salt and black pepper to taste
- <u>Basil Chimichurri:</u>
- 1 ½ cups fresh basil, finely chopped
- 2 banana shallots, diced
- 3 cloves garlic, minced
- 1 tsp red pepper flakes
- ½ cup olive oil
- 3 tbsp red wine vinegar

Directions

Prepare a water bath and place the Sous Vide in it. Set to 140 F. Pat dry the racks with a kitchen towel and rub with pepper and salt. Place meat and garlic in a vacuum-sealable bag, release air by water displacement method and seal the bag. Submerge the bag in the water bath. Set the timer for 2 hours and cook. Make the basil chimichurri: mix all the listed ingredients in a bowl. Cover with cling film and refrigerate for 1 hour 30 minutes. Once the timer has stopped, remove the bag and open it. Remove the lamb and pat dry using a paper towel.

Sear with a torch to a golden brown. Pour the basil chimichurri on the lamb. Serve and enjoy!

CHAPTER 2. Pork

11. Maple Tenderloin with Sautéed Apple

Prep + Cook Time: 2 hours 20 minutes | Servings: 4

Ingredients

- 1 pound pork tenderloin
- 1 tbsp fresh rosemary, chopped
- 1 tbsp maple syrup
- 1 tsp black pepper
- Salt to taste
- 1 tbsp olive oil
- 1 apple, diced
- 1 thinly sliced small shallot
- ¼ cup vegetable broth
- ½ tsp apple cider

Directions

Prepare a water bath and place the Sous Vide in it. Set to 135 F. Remove the skin from the tenderloin and cut by the half. Combine the rosemary, maple syrup, pepper, and salt. Sprinkle over the tenderloin.

Place in a vacuum-sealable bag. Release air by the water displacement method, seal, and submerge the bag in the water bath.

Cook for 2 hours. Once the timer has stopped, remove the bag and dry it. Reserve the cooking juices. Heat olive oil in a skillet over medium heat and sear the tenderloin for 5 minutes. Set aside. Low the heat and put in apple, rosemary springs, and shallot. Season with salt and sauté for 2-3 minutes until golden. Add in vinegar, broth, and cooking juices. Simmer for 3-5 minutes more. Cut the tenderloin into medallions and serve with the apple mix.

12. Balsamic Pork Chops

Prep + Cook Time: 1 hour 15 minutes | Servings: 5

Ingredients

- 2 pounds pork chops
- 3 garlic cloves, crushed
- ½ tsp dried basil
- ½ tsp dried thyme
- ¼ cup balsamic vinegar
- Salt and black pepper to taste
- 3 tbsp extra virgin olive oil

Directions

Prepare a water bath, place Sous Vide in it, and set to 158 F. Season the pork chops generously with salt and pepper; set aside. In a small bowl, combine vinegar with 1 tbsp of olive oil, thyme, basil, and garlic. Stir well and spread the mixture evenly over meat. Place in a large vacuum-sealable bag and seal it.

Submerge the sealed bag in the water bath. Cook for for 1 hour. Once the timer has stopped, take the pork chops out of the bag, and pat them dry. Heat the remaining olive oil in a pan over high heat. Sear the chops for one minute per side, or until golden brown. Add in cooking juices and simmer for 3-4 minutes or until thickened.

Once the timer has stopped, take the bag out, unseal it and remove the ribs. Transfer to a plate and keep it warm. Put a skillet over medium heat and pour in the sauce of the bag. Bring to boil for 5 minutes, reduce the heat, and simmer for 12 minutes. Add the ribs and coat with the sauce. Simmer for 6 minutes. Serve with steamed greens.

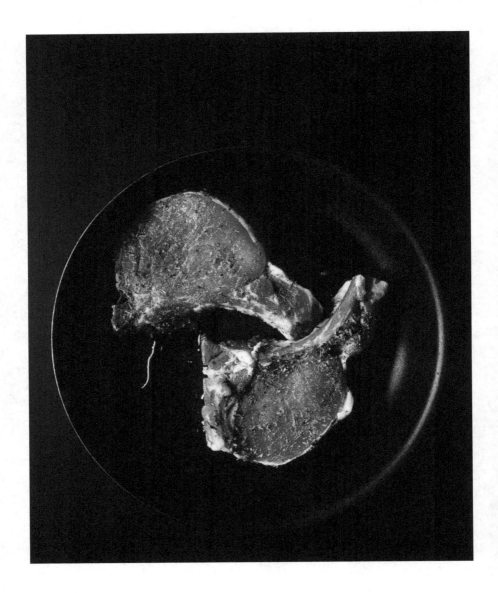

13.Lime and Garlic Pork Tenderloin

Prep + Cook Time: 2 hours 15 minutes | Servings: 2

Ingredients

- 2 tbsp garlic powder
- 2 tbsp ground cumin
- 2 tbsp dried thyme
- 2 tbsp dried rosemary
- 1 pinch lime sea salt
- 2 (3-lb) pork tenderloin, silver skin removed
- 2 tbsp olive oil
- 3 tbsp unsalted butter

Directions

Make a water bath, place Sous Vide in it, and set to 140 F. Add the cumin, garlic powder, thyme, lime salt, rosemary, and lime salt to a bowl and mix evenly. Brush the pork with olive oil and rub with salt and cumin herb mixture. Put the pork into two separate vacuumsealable bags. Release air by the water displacement method and seal the bags. Submerge in the water bath and set the timer for 2 hours.

Once the timer has stopped, remove and unseal the bag. Remove the pork and pat dry using a paper towel. Discard the juice in the bag. Preheat a pan over high heat and add in butter. Place in pork and sear until golden brown, about 4-5 minut. Let the pork rest on a cutting board. Cut them into 2-inch medallions.

14. Flavorful Pork with Mustard & Molasses Glaze

Prep + Cook Time: 4 hours 15 minutes | Servings: 6

Ingredients

- 2 pounds pork loin roast
- 1 bay leaf - 3 oz molasses
- ½ oz soy sauce - ½ oz honey
- Juice of 2 lemons
- 2 strips lemon peel
- 4 chopped scallions
- ½ tsp garlic powder
- ¼ tsp Dijon mustard
- ¼ tsp ground allspice
- 1 oz crushed corn chips

Directions

Prepare a water bath and place the Sous Vide in it. Set to 142 F. Place the pork loin and bay leaf in a vacuum-sealable bag. Add in molasses, soy sauce, lemon peel, honey, scallions, garlic powder, mustard, and allspice; shake well. Release air by the water displacement method, seal, and submerge the bag in the water bath.

Cook for 4 hours. Once the timer has stopped, remove the bag. Pour the remaining mixture into a saucepan and boil until reduced. Serve the pork with the sauce and top with crushed corn chips. Garnish with green onion.

15.Spicy Tenderloin with Sweet Papaya Sauce

Prep + Cook Time: 2 hours 45 minutes | Servings: 4

Ingredients

- ¼ cup light broth sugar
- 1 tbsp ground allspice
- ½ tsp cayenne pepper
- ¼ tsp ground cinnamon
- ¼ tsp ground cloves
- Salt and black pepper to taste
- 2 pounds pork tenderloin
- 2 tbsp canola oil
- 2 pitted and peeled papayas, finely diced
- ¼ cup fresh cilantro, chopped
- 1 red bell pepper, seeded, stemmed and finely diced
- 3 tbsp red onion, finely diced
- 2 tbsp lime juice
- 1 small jalapeno pepper, seeded and diced

Directions

Prepare a water bath and place the Sous Vide in it. Set to 135 F. Combine the sugar, allspice, cinnamon, cayenne, cloves, cumin, salt, and pepper. Sprinkle over the tenderloin.

Heat oil in a skillet over medium heat and sear the tenderloin for 5 minutes. Transfer to a plate and allow resting for 10 minutes. Place in a vacuum-sealable bag. Release air by the water displacement method. Seal and submerge the bag in the water bath. Cook for 2 hours. Once the timer has stopped, remove the tenderloin and allow resting for 10 minutes. Slice them. For the sauce, mix the papaya, cilantro, bell pepper, onion, lime juice, and jalapeño. Serve the tenderloin and top with the sauce. Sprinkle with salt and pepper and serve.

16.Mexican Pork Carnitas with Salsa Roja

Prep + Cook Time: 49 hours 40 minutes | Servings: 8

Ingredients

- 3 tbsp olive oil
- 2 tbsp red pepper flakes
- Salt to taste
- 2 tsp hot Mexican chili powder
- 2 tsp dried oregano
- ½ tsp ground cinnamon
- 2 ¼ pounds boneless pork shoulder
- 4 small ripe tomatoes, diced
- ¼ red onion, diced
- ¼ cup cilantro leaves, chopped
- Freshly squeezed lemon juice
- 8 corn tortillas

Directions

Combine well the red pepper flakes, kosher salt, hot Mexican chili powder, oregano, and cinnamon. Brush chili mix over the pork and cover with aluminium foil. Allow chilling for 1 hour.

Prepare a water bath and place Sous Vide in it. Set to 159 F. Place the pork in a vacuum-sealable bag. Release air by the water displacement method, seal and submerge in the water bath. Cook for 48 hours. 15

minutes Before the end, mix together the tomatoes, onion and cilantro. Add in lemon juice and salt.

Once the timer has stopped, remove the bag and transfer the pork to a cutting board. Discard cooking juices.

Pull the meat until it is shredded. Heat vegetable oil in a skillet over medium heat and cook the shredded pork until it gets crispy and crusty parts. Fill the tortilla with pork. Top with salsa roja and serve.

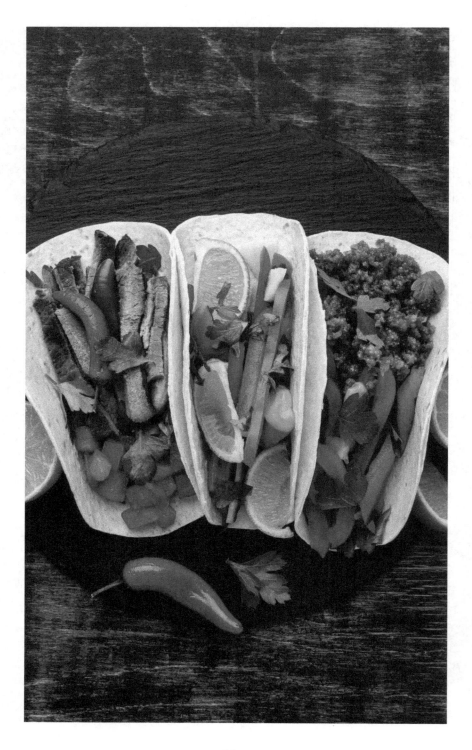

CHAPTER 3.   Poultry

17.Mustard & Garlic Chicken

Prep + Cook Time: 60 minutes | Servings: 5

Ingredients

- 17 ounces chicken breasts
- 1 tbsp Dijon mustard
- 2 tbsp mustard powder
- 2 tsp tomato sauce
- 3 tbsp butter
- 1 tsp salt
- 3 tsp minced garlic ¼ cup soy sauce

Directions

Prepare a water bath and place the Sous Vide in it. Set to 150 F. Place all the ingredients in a vacuum-sealable bag and shake to combine. Release air by the water displacement method, seal, and submerge the bag in the water bath. Set the timer to 50 minutes. Once the timer has stopped, remove the chicken and slice. Serve warm.

18. Yummy Chicken Legs with Lime-Sweet Sauce

Prep + Cook Time: 14 hours 30 minutes | Servings: 8

Ingredients

- ¼ cup olive oil
- 12 chicken legs
- 4 red bell peppers, chopped
- 6 spring onions, chopped
- 4 garlic cloves, minced
- 1 oz fresh ginger, chopped
- ½ cup Worcestershire sauce
- ¼ cup lime juice
- 2 tbsp lime zest
- 2 tbsp sugar
- 2 tbsp fresh thyme leaves
- 1 tbsp allspice
- Salt and black pepper to taste
- 1 tsp ground nutmeg

Directions

Put in a food processor the peppers, onions, garlic, ginger, Worcestershire sauce, olive oil, lime juice and zest, sugar, thyme, allspice, salt, black pepper, and nutmeg. and blend. Reserve 1/4 cup of sauce. Place the chicken and lime sauce in a vacuum-sealable bag. Release air by the water displacement method. Chill for 12 hours. Prepare a water bath and place the Sous Vide in it. Set to 152 F. Seal and submerge the bag in the water bath. Cook for 2 hours. Once the timer has stopped, remove the chicken and pat dry with kitchen towels.

Discard the cooking juices. Brush the chicken with the reserved lime sauce. Heat a skillet over high heat and sear the chicken for 30 seconds per side. Serve and enjoy!

19.Pepper Chicken Salad

Prep + Cook Time: 1 hour 15 minutes | Servings: 4

Ingredients

- 4 chicken breasts, boneless and skinless
- ¼ cup + 3 tbsp vegetable oil
- 1 onion, peeled and finely chopped
- 6 cherry tomatoes, halved
- Salt and black pepper to taste
- 1 cup lettuce, finely chopped
- 2 tbsp freshly squeezed lemon juice

Directions

Make a water bath, place Sous Vide in it, and set to 149 F.

Thoroughly rinse the meat under the cold water and pat dry using a kitchen paper. Cut the meat into bite-sized pieces and place in a vacuum-sealable bag along with ¼ cup of oil and seal. Submerge the bag in the water bath. Once the timer has stopped, remove the chicken from the bag, pat dry and chill at room temperature.

In a bowl, mix the onion, tomatoes, and lettuce. Finally, add the chicken breasts and season with three tablespoons of oil, lemon juice, and salt. Top with Greek yogurt and olives. However, it's optional. Serve cold.

20. Orange Chicken Thighs

Prep + Cook Time: 2 hours | Servings: 4

Ingredients

- 2 pounds chicken thighs
- 2 small chili peppers, finely chopped
- 1 cup chicken broths
- 1 onion, chopped
- ½ cup freshly squeezed orange juice
- 1 tsp orange extract, liquid
- 2 tbsp vegetable oil
- 1 tsp barbecue seasoning mix
- Fresh parsley to garnish

Directions

Make a water bath, place Sous Vide in it, and set to 167 F. Heat olive oil in a large saucepan. Add in chopped onions and stir-fry for 3 minutes, over a medium temperature, until translucent.

In a food processor, combine the orange juice with chili pepper and orange extract. Pulse until well combined. Pour the mixture into a saucepan and reduce the heat. Simmer for 10 minutes. Coat chicken with barbecue seasoning mix and place in a saucepan. Add in chicken broth and cook until half of the liquid evaporates. Remove to a large vacuum-sealable bag and seal. Submerge the bag in the water bath and cook for 45 minutes. Once the timer has stopped, remove the bag and open it. Garnish with fresh parsley and serve.

21.Chicken Stew with Mushrooms

Prep + Cook Time: 1 hour 5 minutes | Servings: 2

Ingredients

- 2 chicken thighs, skinless
- ½ cup fire-roasted tomatoes, diced
- ½ cup chicken stock
- 1 tbsp tomato paste
- ½ cup button mushrooms, chopped
- 1 medium-sized celery stalk
- 1 small carrot, chopped
- 1 small onion, chopped
- 1 tbsp fresh basil, finely chopped
- 1 garlic clove, crushed
- Salt and black pepper to taste

Directions

Make a water bath, place Sous Vide in it, and set to 129 F. Rub the thighs with salt and pepper. Set aside. Chop the celery stalk into halfinch long pieces. Place the meat, onion, carrot, mushrooms, celery stalk, and fire-roasted tomatoes in a vacuum-sealable bag. Submerge the sealed bag in the water bath and set the timer for 45 minutes.

Once the timer has stopped, remove the bag from the water bath and open it. The meat should be falling off the bone easily, so remove the bones. Heat some oil in a medium-sized saucepan and add garlic. Briefly fry for about 3 minutes, stirring constantly. Add the contents of the bag, chicken stock, and tomato paste. Bring it to a boil and reduce the heat to medium. Cook for 5 more minutes, stirring occasionally.

Serve sprinkled with basil.

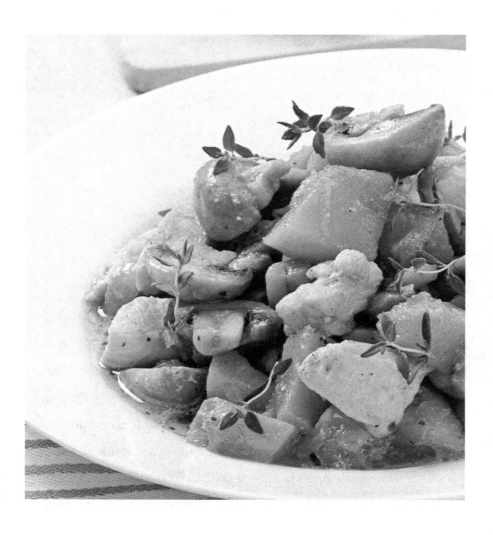

22.   Chicken Thighs with Carrot Puree

Prep + Cook Time: 60 minutes | Servings: 5

Ingredients

- 2 pounds chicken thighs
- 1 cup carrots, pureed
- 2 tbsp olive oil
- ¼ cup finely chopped onion
- 2 cups chicken broth
- 2 tbsp fresh parsley, finely chopped
- 2 crushed garlic cloves
- Salt and black pepper to taste

Directions

Make a water bath, place Sous Vide in it, and set to 167 F. In a bowl, combine 1 tablespoon of olive oil, parsley, salt, and pepper. Stir well and generously brush the thighs with the mixture. Place in a large vacuum-sealable bag and add chicken broth. Press the bag to remove the air. Seal the bag, put it in the water bath, and set the timer to 45 minutes. Once the timer has stopped, remove the thighs from the bag and pat them dry. Reserve the cooking liquid.

Heat the remaining olive oil in a large skillet over medium heat. Add garlic and onion and stir-fry for about 1-2 minutes or until soft. Add chicken thighs and cook for 2-3 minutes, turning occasionally. Taste for doneness, adjust the seasonings and then add broth. Bring it to a boil and remove from the heat. Transfer the thighs to a serving plate. Top with carrot puree and sprinkle with parsley. Serve and enjoy!

23.   Whole Chicken

Prep + Cook Time: 7 hours 15 minutes | Servings:

Ingredients

- 1 (5 lb) full chicken, trussed
- 5 cups chicken stock
- 3 cups mixed bell peppers, diced
- 3 cups celery, diced
- 3 cups leeks, diced
- ¼ tsp salt
- 1 ¼ tsp black peppercorns
- 2 bay leaves

Directions

Make a water bath, place Sous Vide in it, and set to 150 F. Season the chicken with salt. Place all the listed ingredients and chicken in a sizable vacuum-sealable bag. Release air by the water displacement method and seal the vacuum bag. Drop in the water bath and set the timer for 7 hours. Cover the water with a plastic bag to reduce evaporation and water every 2 hours to the bath. Once the timer has stopped, remove and unseal the bag. Preheat a broiler, carefully remove the chicken and pat dry. Place the chicken in the broiler and broil until the skin is golden brown. Rest the chicken for 8 minutes, slice and serve.

24.   Simple Spicy Chicken Thighs

Prep + Cook Time: 2 hours 55 minutes | Servings:

Ingredients

- 1 lb chicken thighs, bone-in
- 3 tbsp butter
- 1 tbsp cayenne pepper
- Salt to taste

Directions

Make a water bath, place Sous Vide in it, and set to 165 F. Season the chicken with pepper and salt. Place chicken with one tablespoon of butter in a vacuum-sealable bag. Release air by the water displacement method, seal, and submerge the bag in the water bath. Set the timer for 2 hours 30 minutes.

Once the timer has stopped, remove the bag and unseal it. Preheat a grill and melt the remaining butter in a microwave.

Grease the grill grate with some of the butter and brush the chicken with the remaining butter. Sear until dark brown color is achieved. Serve as a snack.

25.   Spice Turkey Dish

Prep + Cook Time: 14 hours 15 minutes | Servings: 4

Ingredients

- 1 turkey leg
- 1 tbsp olive oil
- 1 tbsp garlic salt
- 1 tsp black pepper
- 3 sprigs of thyme 1 tbsp rosemary

Directions

Prepare a water bath and place the Sous Vide in it. Set to 146 F. Season the turkey with garlic, salt and pepper.

Place it in a vacuum-sealable bag. Release air by the water displacement method, seal and submerge the bag in the bath. Cook for 14 hours. Once done, remove the legs and pat dry.

CHAPTER 4.   Fish & Seafood

26.   Sous Vide Halibut

Prep + Cook Time: 1 hour 20 minutes | Servings: 4

Ingredients

- 1 pound halibut fillets
- 3 tbsp olive oil
- ¼ cup of shallots, finely chopped
- 1 tsp freshly grated lemon zest
- ½ tsp dried thyme, ground
- 1 tbsp fresh parsley, finely chopped
- 1 tsp fresh dill, finely chopped
- Salt and black pepper to taste

Directions

Wash the fish under cold running water and pat dry with kitchen paper. Cut into thin slices generously sprinkle with salt and pepper. Place in a large vacuum-sealable bag and add two tablespoons of olive oil. Season with shallots, thyme, parsley, dill, salt, and pepper.

Press the bag to remove the air and seal the lid. Shake the bag to coat all fillets with spices and refrigerate for 30 minutes before cooking.

Cook in sous vide for 40 minutes at 131 F. Remove the bag from water and set aside to cool for a while. Place on a kitchen paper and drain. Remove the herbs.

Preheat the remaining oil in a large skillet over high hest. Add fillets and cook for 2 minutes. Flip the fillets and cook for about 35-40 seconds and then remove from the heat. Transfer the fish again to a paper towel and remove excessive fat. Serve immediately.

27.   Sesame Tuna with Ginger Sauce

Prep + Cook Time: 45 minutes | Servings: 6

Ingredients

Tuna:

- 3 tuna steaks
- Salt and black pepper to taste
- ⅓ cup olive oil
- 2 tbsp canola oil
- ½ cup black sesame seeds ½ cup white sesame seeds
- Ginger Sauce:
- 1-inch ginger, grated
- 2 shallots, minced
- 1 red chili, minced
- 3 tbsp water
- 2 ½ lime juice
- 1 ½ tbsp rice vinegar
- 2 ½ tbsp soy sauce
- 1 tbsp fish sauce
- 1 ½ tbsp sugar
- 1 bunch green lettuce leaves

Directions

Start with the sauce: place a small pan over low heat and add olive oil. Once it has heated, add ginger and chili. Cook for 3 minutes. Add sugar and vinegar, stir and cook until sugar dissolves. Add water and bring to a boil. Add in soy sauce, fish sauce, and lime juice and cook for 2 minutes. Set aside to cool.

Make a water bath, place Sous Vide in it, and set to 110 F. Season the tuna with salt and pepper and place in 3 separate vacuumsealable bags. Add olive oil, release air from the bag by the water displacement method, seal, and submerge the bag in the water bath.

Set the timer for 30 minutes.

Once the timer has stopped, remove and unseal the bag. Place tuna aside. Place a skillet over low heat and add canola oil. While heating, mix sesame seeds in a bowl. Pat dry tuna, coat them in sesame seeds and sear top and bottom in heated oil until seeds start to toast. Slice tuna into thin strips. Layer a serving platter with lettuce and arrange tuna on the bed of lettuce. Serve with ginger sauce as a starter.

28.   Mustardy Swordfish

Prep + Cook Time: 55 minutes | Servings : 4

Ingredients

- 2 tbsp olive oil
- 2 swordfish steaks
- Salt and black pepper to taste
- ½ tsp Coleman's mustard
- 2 tsp sesame oil

Directions

Prepare a water bath and place Sous Vide in it. Set to 104 F. Season swordfish with salt and pepper. Mix well the olive oil and mustard. Place the swordfish in a vacuum-sealable bag with the mustard mix. Release air by the water displacement method. Seal and submerge the bag in the water bath. Cook for 30 minutes.

Heat sesame oil in a skillet over high heat. Once the timer has stopped, remove the swordfish and pat dry with kitchen towels. Discard cooking juices. Transfer into the skillet and sear for 30 seconds per side. Cut the swordfish into slices and serve.

29.   Spicy Fish Tortillas

Prep + Cook Time: 35 minutes Servings : 4

Ingredients

- ⅓ cup whipping cream
- 4 halibut fillets, skinned
- 1 tsp chopped fresh cilantro
- ¼ tsp red pepper flakes
- Salt and black pepper to taste
- 1 tbsp cider vinegar
- ½ sweet onion, chopped
- 6 tortillas
- Shredded iceberg lettuce
- 1 large tomato, sliced
- Guacamole for garnish
- 1 lime, quartered

Directions

Prepare a water bath and place the Sous Vide in it. Set to 134 F. Combine fillets with cilantro, red pepper flakes, salt, and pepper. Place in a vacuum-sealable bag. Release air by the water displacement method, submerge the bag in the bath. Cook for 25 minutes.

Meantime, mix the cider vinegar, onion, salt, and pepper. Set aside.

Once the timer has stopped, remove the fillets and pat dry with kitchen towels. Using a blowtorch and sear the fillets. Chop into chunks. Put the fish over the tortilla, add lettuce, tomato, cream, onion mixture and guacamole. Garnish with lime.

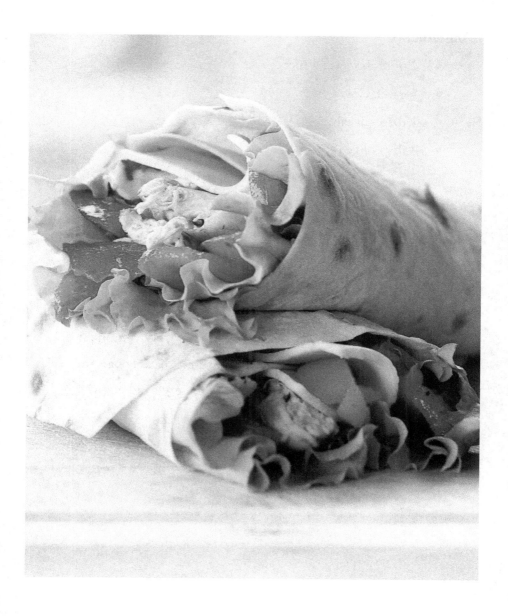

30.   Cilantro Trout

Prep + Cook Time: 60 minutes Servings : 4

Ingredients

- 2 pounds trout, 4 pieces
- 5 garlic cloves
- 1 tbsp sea salt
- 4 tbsp olive oil
- 1 cup cilantro leaves, finely chopped
- 2 tbsp rosemary, finely chopped
- ¼ cup freshly squeezed lemon juice

Directions

Clean and rinse the fish. Pat dry with kitchen paper and rub with salt. Combine garlic with olive oil, cilantro, rosemary, and lemon juice. Use the mixture to fill each fish. Place in a vacuum-sealable bag and seal. Cook en Sous Vide for 45 minutes at 131 F. Serve and enjoy!

31. Tilapia Stew

Prep + Cook Time: 65 minutes Servings : 3

Ingredients

- 1 pound tilapia fillets
- ½ cup onions, finely chopped
- 1 cup carrots, finely chopped
- ½ cup cilantro leaves, finely chopped
- 3 garlic cloves, finely chopped
- 1 cup green bell peppers, chopped
- 1 tsp Italian seasoning mix
- 1 tsp cayenne pepper
- ½ tsp chili pepper
- 1 cup fresh tomato juice
- Salt and black pepper to taste
- 3 tbsp olive oil

Directions

Heat olive oil over medium heat. Add chopped onions and stir-fry until translucent. Now add bell pepper, carrots, garlic, cilantro, Italian seasoning mix, cayenne pepper, chili pepper, salt, and black pepper. Give it a good stir and cook for ten more minutes. Remove from the heat and transfer to a large vacuum-sealable bag along with tomato juice and tilapia fillets. Cook in sous vide for 50 minutes at 122 F. Remove from the water bath and serve.

32.   Basil Tuna Steaks

Prep + Cook Time: 45 minutes Servings : 5

Ingredients

- 6 tbsp olive oil - 4 tuna steaks
- Salt and black pepper to taste
- Zest and juice of 1 lemon
- 2 garlic cloves, minced
- 1 tsp chopped fresh basil

Directions

Prepare a water bath and place Sous Vide in it. Set to 126 F. Season tuna with salt and pepper. Stir 4 tbsp of olive oil, lemon juice and zest, garlic, and basil. Place in two vacuum-sealable bags with the citrus marinate. Release air by the water displacement method, seal and submerge the bags in the water bath. Cook for 35 minutes.

Once the timer has stopped, remove the tuna and pat dry with kitchen towels. Reserve the cooking juices. Heat olive oil in a skillet over high heat and cook the tuna for 1 minute per side. Transfer into a plate and sprinkle with the cooking juices. Best served with rice.

33.   Smoky Salmon

Prep + Cook Time: 1 hour 20 minutes | Servings: 3

Ingredients

- 3 salmon fillets, skinless - 1 tbsp sugar
- 2 tsp smoked paprika
- 1 tsp mustard powder

Directions

Prepare a water bath, place Sous Vide in it, and set it to 115 F. Season the salmon with 1 teaspoon of salt and place in a zipper bag. Refrigerate for 30 minutes. In a bowl, mix the sugar, smoked salt, remaining salt, and mustard powder and mix to combine. Remove the salmon from the fridge and rub with the monk powder mixture. Place salmon in a vacuum-sealable bag, release air by the water displacement method and seal the bag. Submerge in the water bath and set the timer for 45 minutes. Once the timer has stopped, remove the bag and unseal it. Remove the salmon and pat dry using a kitchen towel. Place a non – stick skillet over medium heat, add the salmon and sear it for 30 seconds. Serve with a side of steamed greens.

CHAPTER 5. Eggs

34. Light Vegetarian Frittata

Prep + Cook Time: 1 hour 40 minutes | Servings: 5

Ingredients

- 1 tbsp olive oil
- 1 medium onion, chopped
- Salt to taste
- 4 cloves minced garlic
- 1 daikon - 2 carrots, peeled and diced
- 1 parsnip, peeled and diced
- 1 cup butternut squash, peeled and diced
- 6 oz oyster mushrooms, chopped
- ¼ cup parsley leaves, freshly minced
- A pinch of red pepper flakes
- 5 large eggs - ¼ cup whole milk

Directions

Prepare a water bath and place the Sous Vide in it. Set to 175 F. Grease a few jars with oil. Set aside. Heat a skillet over high heat with oil. Add the onion sweat for 5 minutes. Add garlic and cook for 30 seconds.

Season with salt. Combine carrots, daikon, squash and parsnips. Season with salt and cook 10 minutes more. Add the mushrooms and season with pepper flakes and parsley. Cook for 5 minutes. In a bowl, whisk the eggs and milk Season with salt. Separate the mixture amongst the jars with the vegetables. Seal and submerge the jars in the bath. Cook for 60 minutes. Once ready, remove the jars. Let cool and serve.

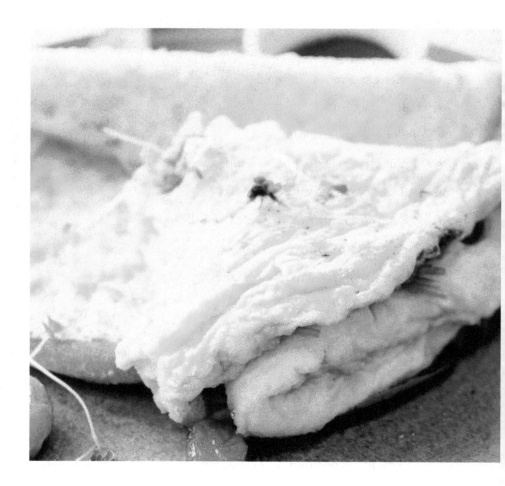

CHAPTER 6. Appetizers and Snacks

35. Carrots & Nuts Stuffed Peppers

Prep + Cook Time: 2 hours 35 minutes | Servings: 5

Ingredients

- 4 shallots, chopped
- 4 carrots, chopped
- 4 garlic cloves, minced
- 1 cup raw cashews, soaked and drained
- 1 cup pecans, soaked and drained
- 1 tbsp balsamic vinegar
- tbsp soy sauce
- 1 tbsp ground cumin
- 2 tsp paprika
- tsp garlic powder
- pinch cayenne pepper
- 4 fresh thyme sprigs
- Zest of 1 lemon
- 4 bell peppers, tops cut off and seeded

Directions

Prepare a water bath and place the Sous Vide in it. Set to 186 F. In a blender, pulse the carrots, garlic, shallots, cashews, pecans, balsamic vinegar, soy sauce, cumin, paprika, garlic powder, cayenne, thyme, and lemon zest.

Pour the mixture into the bell peppers shells and place in a vacuumsealable bag.

Release air by the water displacement method, seal, and submerge the bag in the water bath.

Cook for 1 hour and 15 minutes. Once the timer has stopped, remove the peppers and transfer to a plate.

36.   Easy Spiced Hummus

Prep + Cook Time: 3 hours 35 minutes | Servings: 6

Ingredients

- 1 ½ cups dried chickpeas, soaked overnight
- 2 quarts water
- ¼ cup lemon juice
- ¼ cup tahini paste
- 2 garlic cloves, minced
- 2 tbsp olive oil
- ½ tsp caraway seeds
- ½ tsp salt
- 1 tsp cayenne pepper

Directions

Prepare a water bath and place the Sous Vide in it. Set to 196 F. Strain the chickpeas and place in a vacuum-sealable bag with 1 quart of water. Release air by the water displacement method, seal, and submerge the bag in the water bath. Cook for 3 hours. Once the timer has stopped, remove the bag and transfer into an ice water bath and allow to chill. In a blender, mix the lemon juice and tahini paste for 90 seconds. Add in garlic, olive oil, caraway seeds, and salt, mix for 30 seconds until smooth. Remove the chickpeas and drain it. For a smoother hummus, peel the chickpeas. In a food processor, combine the half of chickpeas with the tahini mix and blend for 90 seconds. Add the remaining chickpeas and blend until smooth. Put the mixture in a plate and garnish with cayenne pepper and the reserved chickpeas.

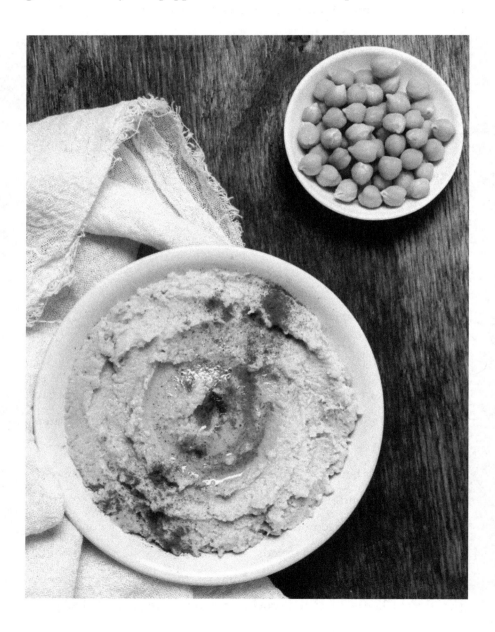

37.   Green Pea Dip

Prep + Cook Time: 45 minutes | Servings: 8

Ingredients

- 2 cups green peas
- 3 tbsp heavy cream
- 1 tbsp tarragon
- 1 tsp olive oil
- Salt and black pepper to taste
- ¼ cup diced apple

Directions

Prepare a water bath and place the Sous Vide in it. Set to 185 F. Place all the ingredients in a vacuum-sealable bag. Release air by the water displacement method, seal, and submerge the bag in the water bath. Set the timer for 32 minutes. Once the timer has stopped, remove the bag and blend with a hand blender until smooth.

38.   Mustard Drumsticks

Prep + Cook Time: 1 hour | Servings: 5

Ingredients

- 2 pounds chicken drumsticks
- ¼ cup Dijon mustard
- 2 garlic cloves, crushed
- 2 tbsp coconut aminos
- 1 tsp pink Himalayan salt
- ½ tsp black pepper

Directions

In a small bowl, combine Dijon with crushed garlic, coconut aminos, salt, and pepper. Spread the mixture over the meat with a kitchen brush and place in a large vacuum-sealable bag. Seal the bag and cook in sous vide for 45 minutes at 167 F. Serve and enjoy!

39.   French Fries

Prep + Cook Time: 45 | Servings: 6

Ingredients

- 3 pounds potatoes, sliced
- 5 cups water
- Salt and black pepper to taste
- ¼ tsp baking soda

Directions

Prepare a water bath and place the Sous Vide in it. Set to 195 F. Place the potato slices, water, salt, and baking soda in a vacuumsealable bag. Release air by the water displacement method, seal, and submerge the bag in the water bath. Set the timer for 25 minutes. Meanwhile, heat the oil in a saucepan over medium heat. Once the timer has stopped, remove the potato slices from the brine and pat dry them. Cook in the oil for a few minutes, until golden.

40.   Stuffed Collard Greens

Prep + Cook Time: 65 minutes | Servings: 3

Ingredients

- 1 pound collard greens, steamed
- 1 pound lean ground beef
- 1 small onion, finely chopped
- 1 tbsp olive oil
- Salt and black pepper to taste
- 1 tsp fresh mint, finely chopped

Directions

Boil a large pot of water and add in greens. Briefly cook, for 2-3 minutes. Drain and gently squeeze the greens and set aside. In a large bowl, combine ground beef, onion, oil, salt, pepper, and mint. Stir well until incorporated. Place leaves on your work surface, vein side up. Use one tablespoon of the meat mixture and place it in the bottom center of each leaf. Fold the sides over and roll up tightly.

Tuck in the sides and gently transfer to a large vacuum-sealable bag. Seal the bag and cook in sous vide for 45 minutes at 167 F.

CHAPTER 7.   Sauces, Stocks and Broths

41.Peri Peri Sauce

Prep + Cook Time: 40 minutes | Servings: 15

Ingredients

- 2 lb red chili peppers
- 4 cloves garlic, crushed
- 2 tsp smoked paprika
- 1 cup cilantro leaves, chopped
- ½ cup basil leaves, chopped
- 1 cup olive oil - 2 lemons' juice

Directions

Make a water bath, place Sous Vide in it, and set to 185 F. Place the peppers in a vacuum-sealable bag. Release air by the water displacement method, seal, and submerge the bag in the water bath. Set the timer for 30 minutes.Once the timer has stopped, remove and unseal the bag. Transfer the pepper and the remaining listed ingredients to a blender and puree to smooth. Store in an airtight container, refrigerate, and use for up to 7 days.

CHAPTER 8.   Vegetarian & Vegan

42.   Lemon Collard Greens Salad with Cranberries

Prep + Cook Time: 15 minutes | Servings: 6

Ingredients

- 6 cups fresh collard greens, stemmed
- 6 tbsp olive oil
- 2 garlic cloves, crushed
- 4 tbsp lemon juice
- ½ tsp salt
- ¾ cup dried cranberries

Directions

Prepare a water bath and place the Sous Vide in it. Set to 196 F. Combine the collard greens with 2 tbsp of olive oil. Place it in a vacuum-sealable bag. Release air by the water displacement method, seal, and submerge the bag in the water bath. Cook for 8 minutes. Stir the remaining olive oil, garlic, lemon juice and salt. Once the timer has stopped, remove the collard greens and transfer onto a serving plate. Sprinkle with the dressing. Garnish with cranberries.

43.　Ginger Tamari Brussels Sprouts with Sesame

Prep + Cook Time: 43 minutes | Servings: 6

Ingredients

- 1 ½ pounds Brussels sprouts, halved
- 2 garlic cloves, minced
- 2 tbsp vegetable oil
- 1 tbsp tamari sauce
- 1 tsp grated ginger
- ¼ tsp red pepper flakes
- ¼ tsp toasted sesame oil
- 1 tbsp sesame seeds

Directions

Prepare a water bath and place Sous Vide in it. Set to 186 F. Heat a pot over medium heat and combine the garlic, vegetable oil, tamari sauce, ginger, and red pepper flakes. Cook for 4-5 minutes. Set aside.

Place the brussels sprouts in a vacuum-sealable bag and pour in tamari mixture. Release air by the water displacement method, seal, and submerge the bag in the water bath. Cook for 30 minutes.

Once the timer has stopped, remove the bag and pat dry with kitchen towels. Reserve the cooking juices. Transfer the sprouts to a bowl and combine with the sesame oil. Plate the sprouts and sprinkle with cooking juices. Garnish with sesame seeds.

44.   Buttered Peas with Mint

Prep + Cook Time: 25 minutes | Servings:

Ingredients

- 1 tbsp butter
- ½ cup snow peas
- 1 tbsp mint leaves, chopped
- A pinch salt
- Sugar to taste

Directions

Make a water bath, place Sous Vide in it, and set to 183 F. Place all the ingredients in a vacuum-sealable bag. Release air by the water displacement method, seal and submerge in the bath. Cook for 15 minutes. Once the timer has stopped, remove and unseal the bag. Transfer the ingredients to a serving plate. Serve as a condiment.

45.   Beet Spinach Salad

Prep + Cook Time: 2 hours 25 minutes | Servings: 3

Ingredients

- ¼ cup beets, trimmed and cut into bite-sized pieces
- 1 cup fresh spinach, chopped
- 2 tbsp olive oil
- tbsp lemon juice, freshly juiced
- 1 tsp balsamic vinegar
- 3 garlic cloves, crushed
- tbsp butter
- Salt and black pepper to taste

Directions

Rinse well and clean beets. Chop into bite-sized pieces and place in a vacuum-sealable bag along with butter and crushed garlic. Cook in Sous Vide for 2 hours at 185 F. Set aside to cool.

Place the spinach in a vacuum-sealable bag and cook in Sous Vide for 10 minutes at 180 F. Remove from the water bath and cool completely. Place in a large bowl and add cooked beets. Season with salt, pepper, vinegar, olive oil, and lemon juice. Serve immediately.

46. Garlic Greens with Mint

Prep + Cook Time: 30 minutes | Servings:

Ingredients

- ½ cup fresh chicory, torn
- ½ cup wild asparagus, finely chopped
- ½ cup Swiss chard, torn
- ¼ cup fresh mint, chopped
- ¼ cup arugula, torn
- 2 garlic cloves, minced
- ½ tsp salt
- 4 tbsp lemon juice, freshly squeezed
- 2 tbsp olive oil

Directions

Fill a large pot with salted water and add greens. Cook for 3 minutes. Remove and drain. Gently squeeze with your hands and then chop the greens. Transfer to a large vacuum-sealable bag and cook in Sous Vide for 10 minutes at 162 F. Remove from the water bath and set aside. Heat olive oil over medium heat in a large skillet. Add garlic and stir-fry for 1 minute. Stir in greens and season with salt. Sprinkle with fresh lemon juice and serve.

47.   Brussel Sprouts in White Wine

Prep + Cook Time: 35 minutes | Servings: 4

Ingredients

- 1 pound Brussels sprouts, trimmed
- ½ cup extra virgin olive oil
- ½ cup white wine
- Salt and black pepper to taste
- 2 tbsp fresh parsley, finely chopped
- 2 garlic cloves, crushed

Directions

Place Brussels sprouts in a large vacuum-sealable bag with three tablespoons of olive oil. Cook in Sous Vide for 15 minutes at 180 F. Remove from the bag.

In a large, non-stick grill pan, heat the remaining olive oil. Add Brussels sprouts, crushed garlic, salt, and pepper. Briefly grill, shaking the pan a couple of times until lightly charred on all sides. Add wine and bring it to a boil. Stir well and remove from the heat. Top with finely chopped parsley and serve.

48.   Cauliflower Broccoli Soup

Prep + Cook Time: 70 minutes | Servings:

Ingredients

- 1 head cauliflower, cut into florets
- ½ lb broccoli, cut into small florets
- 1 green bell pepper, chopped
- 1 onion, diced
- 1 tsp olive oil
- 1 clove garlic, crushed ½ cup vegetable stock - ½ cup skimmed milk

Directions

Make a water bath, place the Sous Vide in it, and set it to 185 F. Place the cauliflower, broccoli, bell pepper, and white onion in a vacuumsealable bag and pour olive oil into it. Release air by the water displacement method and seal the bag. Submerge the bag in the water bath. Set the timer for 50 minutes and cook.

Once the timer has stopped, remove the bag and unseal. Transfer the vegetables to a blender, add garlic and milk, and puree to smooth. Place a pan over medium heat, add the vegetable puree and vegetable stock and simmer for 3 minutes. Season with salt and pepper. Serve warm as a side dish.

49.   Bell Pepper Puree

Prep + Cook Time: 40 minutes | Servings: 4

Ingredients

- 8 red bell peppers, cored
- ⅓ cup olive oil - 2 tbsp lemon juice
- 3 cloves garlic, crushed
- 2 tsp sweet paprika

Directions

Make a water bath and place Sous Vide in it and set to 183 F. Put the bell peppers, garlic, and olive oil in a vacuum-sealable bag. Release air by the water displacement method, seal and submerge the bags in the water bath. Set the timer for 20 minutes and cook. Once the timer has stopped, remove the bag and unseal.

Transfer the bell pepper and garlic to a blender and puree to smooth. Place a pan over medium heat; add bell pepper puree and the remaining ingredients. Cook for 3 minutes. Serve warm or cold as a dip.

50.   Radish with Herb Cheese

Prep + Cook Time: 1 hour 15 minutes | Servings: 3

Ingredients

- 10 oz goat cheese
- 4 oz cream cheese
- ¼ cup red bell pepper, minced
- 3 tbsp pesto
- 3 tsp lemon juice
- 2 tbsp parsley
- 2 clove garlic
- 9 large radishes, sliced.

Directions

Make a water bath, place Sous Vide in it, and set to 181 F.Place the radish slices in a vacuum-sealable bag, release air and seal it. Submerge the bag in the water bath and set the timer for 1 hour. In a bowl, mix the remaining listed ingredients and pour the mixture into a piping bag. Set aside. Once the timer has stopped, remove the bag and unseal. Arrange the radish slices on a serving platter and pipe the cheese mixture on each slice. Serve as a snack.

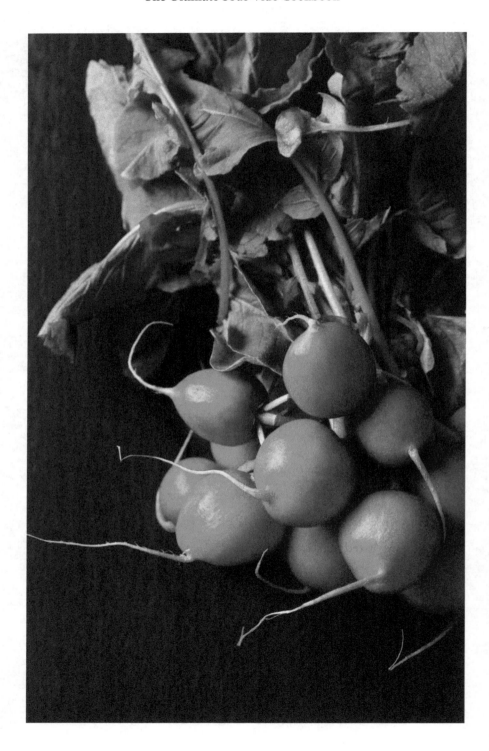

CHAPTER 9.   Desserts & Drinks

51.Easy Banana Cream

Prep + Cook Time: 60 minutes | Servings: 6

Ingredients

- 3 banans, mashed
- 12 egg yolks
- 1 cup superfine sugar
- 3 cups heavy cream
- 1 tsp vanilla extract
- 1 tsp mint extract

Directions

Prepare a water bath and place the Sous Vide in it. Set to 196 F. With an electric mixer, combine the egg yolks and sugar. Mix for 1-2 minutes until creamy. Heat the cream in a saucepan over medium heat and add in vanilla and mint. Cook on Low for 3-4 minutes. Set aside and allow to cool for 2-3 minutes.

Once the mixture has cooled, pour the cream mixture into the egg mixture and stir. Add in mashed bananas and stir to combine. Pour the mixture into 6 mini mason jars. Seal and submerge in the water bath. Cook for 45 minutes. Once the timer has stopped, remove the jars and allow to cool for 5 minutes.

52.　　Apple Pie

Prep + Cook Time: 85 minutes | Servings: 8

Ingredients

- 1 pound apples, peel and cubed
- 6 ounces puff pastry
- 1 egg yolk, whisked
- 4 tbsp sugar
- 2 tbsp lemon juice
- tbsp cornstarch
- 1 tsp ground ginger
- 2 tbsp butter, melted
- ¼ tsp nutmeg
- ¼ tsp cinnamon

Directions

Preheat your oven to 365 F. Roll the pastry into a circle. Brush with the butter and place in the oven. Cook for 15 minutes. Prepare a water bath and place Sous Vide in it. Set to 160 F. Combine all the remaining ingredients in a vacuum-sealable bag. Release air by water displacement method, seal and submerge in the water bath.

Cook for 45 minutes. Once the timer has stopped, remove the bag. Top the cooked pie crust with the apple mixture. Return to the oven and cook for 15 more minutes.

53.　　Dulce de Leche Cheesecake

Prep + Cook Time: 5 hours 55 minutes + 4 hours | Servings: 6

Ingredients

- 2 cups mascarpone,softened
- 3 eggs - 1 tsp almond extract
- 1 cup dulce de leche
- ⅓ cup heavy cream
- 1 cup graham cracker crumbs
- 3 tbsp butter, melted
- ½ tsp salt

Directions

Prepare a water bath and place the Sous Vide in it. Set to 175 F. With an electric mixer, mix the mascarpone, eggs, and almond in a bowl until smooth. Pour 3/4 cup of dulce de leche and mix well. Add in cream and stir until fully combined. Set aside. Combine the graham cracker crumbs and melted butter. Divide the crumbs mixture into six mini mason jars. Pour cream cheese mixture over the crumbs. Seal with a lid and submerge the jars in the water bath. Cook for 1 hour and 30 minutes. Once the timer has stopped, remove the jars and transfer into the fridge and allow to cool for 4 hours. Top with the remaining dulce de leche. Garnish with the salted caramel mixture.

54. Sugar-Free Chocolate Chip Cookies

Prep + Cook Time: 3 hours 45 minutes | Servings: 6

Ingredients

- 1/3 cup chocolate chips
- 7 tbsp heavy cream
- 2 eggs - ½ cup flour
- ½ tsp baking soda
- 4 tbsp butter, melted - ¼ tsp salt
- 1 tbsp lemon juice

Directions

Prepare a water bath and place the Sous Vide in it. Set to 194 F. Beat the eggs along with the cream, lemon juice, salt, and baking soda. Stir in flour and butter. Fold in the chocolate chips.

Divide the dough between 6 ramekins. Wrap them well with plastic foil and place the ramekins in the water bath. Cook for 3 hours and 30 minutes. Once the timer has stopped, remove the ramekins.

55.   Raisin-Stuffed Sweet Apples

Prep + Cook Time: 2 hours 15 minutes | Servings: 4

Ingredients

- 4 small apples, peeled and cored
- 1 ½ tbsp raisins
- 4 tbsp butter, softened
- ¼ tsp nutmeg
- ½ tsp cinnamon 1 tbsp sugar

Directions

Prepare a water bath and place the Sous Vide in it. Set to 170 F. Combine the raisins, sugar, butter, cinnamon, and nutmeg. Stuff the apples with the raisin mixture. Divide the apples between 2 vacuumsealable bag Release air by the water displacement method, seal and submerge the bags in the water bath. Set the timer for 2 hours. Once the timer has stopped, remove the bags. Serve warm.

56. Bread Pudding

Prep + Cook Time: 2 hours 15 minutes | Servings: 8

Ingredients

- 1 cup milk
- 1 cup heavy cream
- 10 ounces white bread
- 4 eggs
- 2 tbsp butter, melted
- 1 tbsp flour
- 1 tbsp cornstarch
- 4 tbsp sugar
- 1 tsp vanilla extract
- ¼ tsp salt

Directions

Prepare a water bath and place the Sous Vide in it. Set to 170 F. Chop the bread into small pieces and place in a vacuum-sealable bag. Beat the eggs along with the remaining ingredients. Pour the mixture over the bread. Release air by the water displacement method, seal, and submerge the bag in the water bath. Set the timer for 2 hours. Once the timer has stopped, remove the bag. Serve warm.

57. Rice Pudding with Rum & Cranberries

Prep + Cook Time: 2 hours 15 minutes | Servings: 6

Ingredients

- 2 cups rice - 3 cups milk
- ½ cup dried cranberries soaked in ½ cup of rum overnight and drained
- 1 tsp cinnamon - ½ cup brown sugar

Directions

Prepare a water bath and place the Sous Vide in it. Set to 140 F. Combine all the ingredients in a bowl and transfer to 6 small jars. Seal them and submerge in the water bath. Set the timer for 2 hours. Once the timer has stopped, remove the jars. Serve warm or chilled.

58. Lemon Curd

Prep + Cook Time: 75 minutes | Servings: 8

Ingredients

- 1 cup butter
- 1 cup sugar
- 12 egg yolks 5 lemons

Directions

Prepare a water bath and place the Sous Vide in it. Set to 168 F.

Grate the zest from lemons and place in a bowl. Squeeze the juice and add to the bowl as well. Whisk on the yolks and sugar and transfer to a vacuum-sealable bag. Release air by the water displacement method, seal, and submerge the bag in the water bath. Set the timer for 1 hour. Once the timer has stopped, remove the bag and transfer the cooked lemon curd to a bowl and place in an ice bath. Let chill completely.

59.   Crème Brulee

Prep + Cook Time: 45 minutes | Servings: 4

Ingredients

- 2 cups heavy cream
- 4 egg yolks
- ¼ cup sugar
- 1 tsp vanilla extract

Directions

Prepare a water bath and place the Sous Vide in it. Set to 180 F. Whisk together all the ingredients and transfer into 4 shallow jars.Seal and immerse in the water bath. Cook for 30 minutes. Once the timer has stopped, remove the shallow jars and sprinkle some sugar on top of the brulee. Place under broiler until they become caramelized.

60.   Spicy Agave Liquor

Prep + Cook Time: 55 minutes | Servings: 8

Ingredients

- 2 cups vodka - ½ cup water
- ½ cup light agave nectar
- 3 dried Guajillo chili peppers
- 1 jalapeno pepper, halved and seeded
- 1 Fresno pepper, halved and seeded
- Zest of 1 lemon
- 1 cinnamon stick
- 1 tsp black peppercorns

Directions

Prepare a water bath and place the Sous Vide in it. Set to 182 F. Combine all the ingredients and place in a vacuum-sealable bag. Release air by the water displacement method, seal, and submerge the bag in the water bath. Cook for 45 minutes. Once the timer has stopped, remove the bag and drain the contents. Allow chilling.